CONTENTS

CENTRAL VENOUS LINES

WHO MAY HAVE A CENTRAL VENOUS CATHETER?

- Any patient who has long-term need of access to a venous route and administration for medication, nutrients or for blood sampling.

- Children with malignant disease who return home with a central venous catheter in place, so that they are not subjected to repeated venepuncture.

GENERAL INFORMATION

- A Hickman line is one type of central venous catheter. It is tunnelled beneath the skin in order to reduce the risk of infection associated with central venous lines and is the one most commonly used in the UK. The literature from the USA might mention Groshong catheters or implanted ports, both of which are similar devices, but the port is implanted beneath the skin with a catheter leading to the central veins.

- The Hickman catheter is a flexible silicone tube about 90cm long which is inserted through a large vein and usually into the vena cava. The external end is capped with an injectable cap and a dressing covers the point of entry. It has a small roughened cuff at the point of entry which sets up an inflammatory reaction, causing fibrosis of the surrounding tissue, and it is this which holds the catheter in place.

- A Hickman catheter can remain in place for up to two years. It does not require intravenous infusion to remain patent but will require regular flushing in order to prevent blockage.

- Hickman lines are frequently used to administer drugs or nutrients to patients receiving treatment for cancer. Such treatment is often immunosuppressive, and it is therefore vital that no infection is introduced either during insertion or maintenance of the catheter.

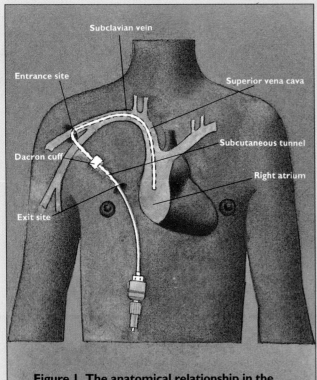

Figure 1. The anatomical relationship in the placement of a tunnelled central venous catheter

INSERTION OF A CENTRAL VENOUS LINE

- A central venous line will normally be inserted under general anaesthetic in the operating room under sterile conditions. The line can also be inserted under a local anaesthetic.

- The operative procedure involves a subclavicular incision and identification of the subclavian vein. A tunnel is made, between the skin and the chest wall, from the incision to the lower chest wall and a second incision made. One end of the catheter is then pulled through the tunnel until the Dacron roughened cuff is at the opening of the second incision. This exit site incision is then sutured and the end of the catheter fitted with an injectable cap.

- An incision is made in the subclavian vein and the tip of the catheter is threaded along the vein, through the superior vena cava and may go into the right atrium.[1] Once the catheter is correctly positioned, the subclavicular incision is sutured.

- All sutures can be removed after eight to 10 days, when the catheter will be held in place by the fibrosed tissue around the roughened cuff.

- Check that the tip is in the correct position with an X-ray before use.

REFERENCE
[1] Pritchard, A.P., David, J.A. (eds). *Royal Marsden Hospital Manual of Nursing Procedures*. London: Harper and Row, 1988..

NURSING THE PATIENT WITH A HICKMAN LINE

■ Patients discharged from hospital with a Hickman line *in situ* will usually have been taught how to dress and flush the catheter. If patients are unable to do this for themselves (for instance, children), relatives or friends can be instructed in daily care. However, continued support and monitoring will be needed at home, and any community nurse who will be involved in caring for a patient with a Hickman line should make arrangements to have a course of instruction and period of familiarisation with this device. This is probably best done in hospital, perhaps in the ward where the patient is being treated before discharge.

■ The exit site must be dressed each day for the first 10 days. After that, it needs dressing only if the site has become infected. Even if the patient has been taught how to do this, it is advisable for the nurse to watch this procedure, as it may be necessary for the nurse to reinforce what has already been taught, perhaps on more than one occasion, so that the patient acquires a good technique and gains confidence.

■ When it is not being used, the catheter should be flushed regularly (one hospital recommends flushing with heparin three times a week, but local policies on this may differ and should be checked). As with dressings, the patient will probably have been taught to do this in hospital, but it is useful for the nurse to check how the procedure is managed in the home surroundings and help the patient become confident.

■ The catheter should also be flushed after it has been used for blood sampling. This helps prevent it becoming blocked. If heparin is used for flushing, the first 10ml of blood should be discarded.

■ The incision site should be checked each day (by patient or nurse) for redness, swelling or exudate which could indicate an infection. This should always be reported either to the hospital or the GP.

■ If the cap has to be changed, the catheter must be clamped to prevent haemorrhage or air being sucked in through the tube because of negative central venous pressure. Aseptic technique should be used.

■ If there is any resistance to flushing from the catheter, it may indicate a blockage. Do not try to flush this through but contact the hospital straight away for further advice.

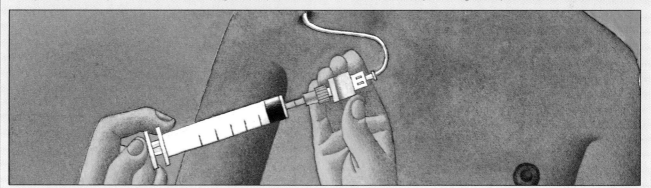

ADVICE TO THE PATIENT

■ Aspects of self-care of the catheter have already been outlined. It is important that both the patient and his or her carers are confident about their ability to manage catheters and feel competent to perform the care required of them.

■ Patients can shower or bath with the catheter *in situ* and should change the dressing afterwards. Waterproof transparent dressings may be used which do not need to be changed.

■ Swimming cannot be allowed because of the risk of infection.

■ Clamps should be carried at all times by the patient, with a spare cap, in case the catheter starts to leak or is damaged. The patient should be instructed to apply the clamps between herself or himself and the damaged part of the catheter.

■ Patients should be taught to recognise signs of infection of the wound site and to report them immediately to the hospital or GP.

■ It should be pointed out to the patient that any resistance to the flow when flushing the catheter could indicate that the catheter is blocked, and this, too, should be reported to the hospital or GP.

AFTER READING THIS YOU SHOULD:

■ Be aware of the nursing skills involved in caring for a patient with a central venous line *in situ*

■ Be aware of the information that patients and carers need to manage self-care of a central venous catheter.

Nurses should be aware of local policies regarding the care of patients with central venous catheters and should liaise with the hospital where the patient has been treated. For further instruction in the practical skills required, contact your local community tutor or an oncology nurse specialist.

FURTHER READING
Conroy, C.S. Groshong catheter or implanted port: which is best for you? *Oncology Nursing Forum* 1990; **17**: 5.
Pike, S. Family participation in the care of central venous lines. *Nursing* 1989; **3**: 38.

SUPPORTING THE PATIENT WITH ASTHMA

GENERAL INFORMATION

■ Most people with asthma can be treated successfully in the community. However, recent evidence suggests that asthma remains underdiagnosed and often ineffectively managed, so that both adults and children have poorly controlled asthma, leading to acute episodes and, in some cases, hospital admission.

■ The effective management of asthma relies not only on adequate clinical assessment and treatment by doctors and nurses but on knowledgeable self-management by the patient. It is particularly important that people with asthma are involved in their own treatment. For prophylactic therapy to be effective, the patient has to use the treatment regularly in the absence of symptoms; he or she must understand thoroughly its importance and must know how to use the inhaler devices. The importance of patient education cannot be over-emphasised.

■ The care of people with asthma demands a well-coordinated team approach so that people can be offered the most appropriate care for their needs at any one time and so that the advice and information they are given is consistent. For this reason it is helpful to construct a protocol to guide a team in caring for people with asthma.

■ This update is a companion to that in Skills Update 1 in which the diagnosis and treatment of asthma were reviewed.

THE DIAGNOSIS OF ASTHMA

■ Confirmation of the diagnosis will be done by a medical practitioner, but, because many cases of asthma still go unrecognised, it is important that nurses are able to identify symptoms indicating asthma.

■ Anyone with recurrent wheezy chest conditions may have asthma: this includes children, who may present with frequent chest infections resulting in a wheeze. In addition, asthma should be suspected in adults and children who have a nocturnal cough or poor exercise tolerance.

■ Early morning wheeze, or tightness of the chest, may be attributable to asthma.

■ Children who have hay-fever or eczema may have accompanying asthma.

■ Measuring the peak expiratory flow rate (PEFR) can demonstrate air-flow limitation. If the PEFR is near normal in the surgery, it is worth asking the patient to carry out measurements at home, to be done in the mornings and the evenings and after exercise. This can demonstrate either diurnal or exercise-provoked variations typical of asthma.

■ If the PEFR shows air-flow limitation, an inhaled bronchodilator may reverse this. If it does, bronchoconstriction is suggested and indicates asthma. The test can be conducted by a medical practitioner or a nurse with special training in the management of asthma.

CONSTRUCTING PROTOCOLS

■ A protocol is a useful way of setting out a team's expectation of the standard of care they will give and who is doing what. It can also establish how and when things are to be done.

■ A protocol constructed by all those involved in the care of a patient with asthma can help to ensure that the condition is properly diagnosed and treated and that patients are not lost to follow-up. It should ideally include the following points:

— What are its aims and objectives? This is the standard at which the practice is aiming. The aim may be something like 'to ensure that all patients with asthma are identified and that their condition is adequately controlled'. The objectives should set out how that aim is to be achieved and should therefore be measurable.

— How will patients with asthma be identified? Will there be opportunistic screening of all those with wheezy chest symptoms, for example? Exact methods should be specified, together with who is to do the screening.

— Once patients are identified, what will be done at their initial assessment, and who will do it?

— At what intervals will they be followed up? Who will be responsible?

— Will the practice keep a register of which patients have asthma? If so, who will enter the patient's name in that register? At what stage will that be done?

— Who can alter the medication, and what treatment regime is acceptable to all in the practice? If a nurse is adequately trained in the care of patients with asthma she should be able to alter treatment regimes by protocol.

— When should patients be referred to the doctor or to the hospital? This may depend on the results of a PEFR test or on the presentation of other symptoms, but it is important to specify these points.

— Where will records be kept? This may be especially important if some care or advice is given by a nurse who is attached to the practice and who keeps other records. What should be noted in the records? Does the patient carry a record, and what is the function of this in treatment and education?

— How will patients be followed up? What will happen if they default on appointments, and who is responsible then for initiating new appointments?

— How will this protocol be evaluated? It provides a standard of care, which can be audited. Who will do it?

GUIDELINES FOR THE MANAGEMENT OF ASTHMA

■ The goal in treating asthma is to allow people with the condition to live as normal a life as possible with the highest possible level of activity they desire.

■ Patient education is crucial if treatment is to be adhered to and properly administered. It is therefore important to find out patients' beliefs about the condition and what their fears may be as a prelude to management. If, for example, patients believe that inhaled medication has to be swallowed to be effective, that will preclude success with inhaled medication until the belief is corrected.

■ Subjects that should be addressed include when to take medication, how to use inhaler devices and what to do when symptoms worsen. It is now possible to prescribe peak flow meters for patients with asthma so they can be taught to monitor their condition with some accuracy and to increase their treatment appropriately. In addition, they can be taught when they should contact their doctor or go to the hospital. This can be particularly reassuring for parents, who can be frightened by asthma symptoms in their children.

■ Drugs used in the treatment of asthma have two main functions: to reduce inflammatory changes in the airways and to relieve bronchospasm.

■ It is now recommended that anti-inflammatory drugs are introduced into the treatment of asthma at a much earlier stage than was once thought desirable. If a bronchodilator has to be used more than once a day, or patients have night-time symptoms, a prophylactic anti-inflammatory drug should be introduced.

■ The most commonly used group of bronchodilator drugs are the β_2 agonists, which act by stimulating the β_2 receptors in the lungs and causing bronchodilation. β_2 agonist drugs can usually be successfully administered by inhalation, and patients should take them as required.

■ If the bronchodilator is required more than once a day, an anti-inflammatory drug should be introduced. The British Thoracic Society guidelines for adult management recommend that a corticosteroid is the drug of first choice at this stage.

■ Steroidal and non-steroidal anti-inflammatory drugs can be given by inhaler and must be taken regularly, even in the absence of symptoms, to be effective.

■ If asthma is not well controlled on this regime, a higher dose of steroids can be introduced, perhaps administered by a spacer device such as a Volumatic (see Skills Update 1). It is not thought that even the long-term use of steroid drugs in the control of asthma carries a significant risk to the patient from side-effects. To minimise the amount of steroid drug swallowed when using an inhalation device, patients can be instructed to wash out their mouths after treatment.

■ If symptom relief is still inadequate, a long-acting inhaled bronchodilator may be used or an oral β_2 agonist, in addition to other medication.

■ Oral steroid therapy may be considered for maintenance therapy if other measures are still inadequate.

■ The aim of treatment should be to provide effective control with the minimum amount of drug therapy. Treatment therefore has to be flexible, with regular reviews of the individual patient's condition.

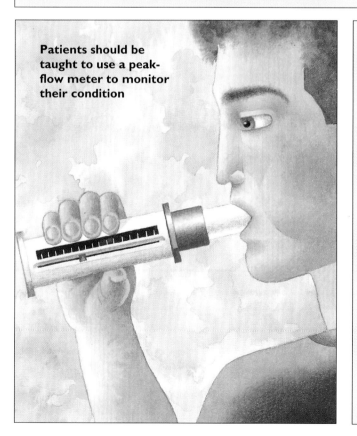

Patients should be taught to use a peak-flow meter to monitor their condition

NOW YOU SHOULD BE AWARE OF:

■ The signs and certain recurring symptoms suggesting an asthmatic condition and know when to refer to a medical practitioner for further screening

■ The correct way to approach patient education on the principles of asthma treatment

■ How to construct a protocol with others for the care of people with asthma.

Specialised training courses for nurses are offered at the Asthma Training Centre, Winton House, Church Street, Stratford-upon-Avon CV37 6HB.

FURTHER READING
British Thoracic Society, Royal College of Physicians of London, King's Fund Centre, National Asthma Campaign. Guidelines for the management of asthma in adults: 1. Chronic persistent asthma. *British Medical Journal* 1990; 301: 651–653.
British Thoracic Society, Royal College of Physicians of London. King's Fund Centre, National Asthma Campaign. Guidelines for the management of asthma in adults: 2. Acute severe asthma. *British Medical Journal* 1990; 301: 797–800.
Pearson, R. *Asthma Management in Primary Care*. Oxford: Radcliffe Medical Press, 1990.

ELECTROCARDIOGRAMS

WHY RECORD AN ECG?

- The electrocardiogram (ECG) records the electrical activity of the heart. It is therefore possible to identify such disorders as conduction abnormalities, damage to the myocardium and cardiac dysrhythmias from an ECG tracing.
- An ECG is an aid to the diagnosis of a number of heart problems, and it is likely that it will be a procedure carried out on patients who have symptoms attributable to cardiac disorders.
- Because it is an aid to diagnosis, it is important that the ECG is recorded as accurately as possible.

PHYSIOLOGICAL CONSIDERATIONS

- It is necessary to understand the conduction system of the heart in order to understand what the ECG is recording. What follows is a summary of the electrical structure of the heart. For more information you should read a physiology textbook.
- Electrical activity in the heart precedes mechanical activity. It is an electrical impulse that causes the heart to contract, and it is this myocardial function which results in a pulse. In a healthy heart the electrical and mechanical activity will be integrated so that each electrical impulse corresponds with a pulse.
- Heart cells have four properties which allow for the integration of electrical and mechanical activity:
  – Automaticity: the ability to initiate electrical impulses
  – Excitability: the ability to respond to electrical stimuli
  – Conductivity: the ability to transmit electrical impulses
  – Contractility: the ability to respond to electrical impulses by contracting — the pump action.
- Electrical stimulation at the heart begins in the sinoatrial node, located in the wall of the right atrium, close to the superior vena cava. The sinoatrial node is the normal pacemaker of the heart, because it initiates impulses at a faster rate than other areas of the heart. The characteristic rate of sinoatrial node stimulation (about 70 beats a minute) is called sinus rhythm.
- The autonomic nervous system influences the sinoatrial node and can cause the heart rate to increase (sympathetic effect) or decrease (parasympathetic effect). However, the automaticity of the sinoatrial node means that even if separated from the auto-nomic nervous system it can initiate its own electrical activity.
- Once an electrical impulse is sent out by the sinoatrial node it can travel throughout the heart because of the conductive properties of the cardiac cells. This is possible because of a process called depolarisation. A cell receiving an electrical stimulus is negatively charged (polarised). In order to transmit the electrical stimulus it must become positively charged, and it is then depolarised. Having transmitted the charge, the cell once again becomes negatively charged (repolarisation) ready to receive the next impulse. The wave of depolarisation and repolarisation is what the ECG can detect and record.
- From the sinoatrial node the depolarisation wave spreads through conduction tissue in the atria, causing them to contract. It then reaches the atrioventricular node where it is delayed for about 0.1 of a second to allow the completion of atrial contraction. From the atrioventricular node the impulse spreads rapidly through the atrioventricular bundle (Bundle of His) and the bundle branches in the ventricular septum, finally reaching the Purkinje fibres in the ventricular myocardium. The total time elapsing between the initiation of the impulse by the sinoatrial node and depolarisation of the last of the ventricular muscle cells is 0.22 seconds in the healthy adult heart.
- Ventricular contraction follows the ventricular depolarisation wave.

THE MEANING OF THE ECG TRACING

- The changes in cell charges which occur during depolarisation and repolarisation can be recorded with an ECG. The cell changes produce waves or deflections on the ECG recording paper. This occurs because the electrical currents generated by, and transmitted through, the heart also spread through the body, transmitted by body fluids.
- The typical ECG shows three waves: these are known as the P wave, the QRS complex and the T wave.
- The P wave results from atrial depolarisation — that is, the impulse conduction from the sinoatrial node through the atria.
- The QRS complex results from ventricular depolarisation. The two waves in the QRS complex show depolarisation through both the differently sized ventricles.
- The T wave results from the repolarisation of the ventricles. The atria repolarise during the QRS wave, but the electrical activity caused by atrial repolarisation is too weak to be recorded.
- The size, duration and timing of the P, QRS and T waves tend to be consistent in a healthy heart. Changes in the timing of the waves, or in their pattern, usually indicate damage to the myocardial cells, so that they can no longer depolarise and repolarise (as in a myocardial infarct), or to the heart's conduction system (for example, in heart block).

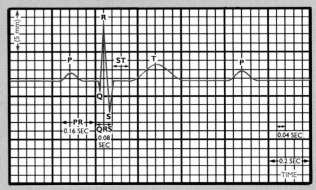

The basic features of an ECG

THE INTRINSIC CONDUCTION SYSTEM OF THE HEART

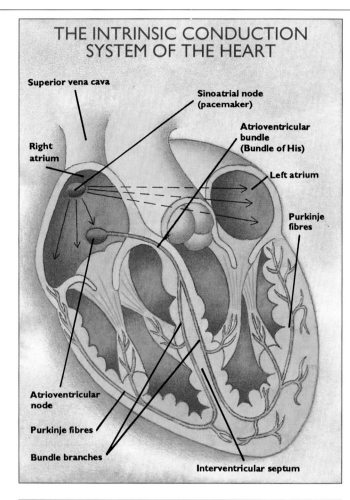

Superior vena cava

Sinoatrial node (pacemaker)

Atrioventricular bundle (Bundle of His)

Right atrium

Left atrium

Purkinje fibres

Atrioventricular node

Purkinje fibres

Bundle branches

Interventricular septum

NURSING CONSIDERATIONS IN TAKING AN ECG

- Some patients are afraid that the ECG procedure could electrocute them. Explain that this is not so and that they will feel no discomfort during the test.
- The electrode must make good contact with the skin. A special gel can be used, but it might be necessary to shave a small area on a very hairy chest. Avoid the hairiest parts of limbs.
- Even the slightest movement can reduce the quality of an ECG tracing. Explain to the patient why it is necessary to lie still and not to talk during the procedure.
- Some ECGs are taken while the patient is exercising so that the effect of physical activity on chest pain, cardiac dysrhythmias and other cardiac symptoms can be determined. Exercise ECGs are also useful to gauge recovery after myocardial infarct. For an exercise ECG the patient should not smoke or eat for two hours before the procedure, as this can distort the results. Comfortable shoes and loose-fitting clothes should be worn. Explain that the exercise will make the patient perspire and that the heart rate will increase. Explain that the ECG recording will end when the heart rate has reached a predetermined level. Reassure the patient that the exercise can be stopped immediately if he or she experiences chest pain, breathlessness, severe fatigue or leg pain. While the investigation is in progress the patient should be observed for any signs of exercise intolerance.

HOW THE ECG MACHINE WORKS

- The ECG uses two different methods to record the electrical activity of the heart. The first is by the use of bi-polar leads. A bi-polar lead uses two electrodes, one positive and one negative, and the ECG machine traces the electric current passing between them.
- There are three bi-polar leads: one is placed on the right arm, one on the left arm and the other on the left leg. In the two arm positions, the left arm lead is made positive and the right negative. The reading of the current between the two positions is called lead I. Lead II traces the current between the right arm (negative) and left leg (positive), and lead III is the current between the left arm (now made negative) and the left leg (positive).
- The electrode attached to the right leg is a neutralising electrode only, so that the electrode on the left leg acts as the major foot electrode.
- The second way in which the ECG machine records electric impulses is by using positively charged electrodes alone. These are called unipolar leads. Nine unipolar leads are commonly used, three on the limbs as before and six positioned on the chest wall (V leads). Because the electrical forces recorded by a unipolar lead are small, this system must use augmented voltage, and hence these leads are called aV (augmented voltage). The initials R, L and F refer to the electrode sites: R is right arm, L is left arm and F is foot (left leg).
- Each lead of the ECG machine views the heart from a different angle. The following table shows the views obtained by a 12-lead ECG.

Lead	View of heart	Lead	View of heart
I	Lateral wall	V_1	Anteroseptal wall
II	Inferior wall	V_2	Anteroseptal wall
III	Inferior wall	V_3	Anterior wall
aVR	No specific view	V_4	Anterior wall
aVL	Lateral wall	V_5	Lateral wall
aVF	Inferior wall	V_6	Lateral wall

NOW YOU SHOULD FEEL COMPETENT TO:

- Understand what an ECG is recording
- Recognise a normal ECG tracing
- Reassure a patient undergoing an ECG.

FURTHER READING
Hampton, J. *The ECG Made Easy*. Edinburgh: Churchill Livingstone, 1985.
Marieb, E. *Human Anatomy and Physiology*. California: Benjamin/Cummings Publishing Company, 1989.
Ortiz Vinsant, M., Spence, M. *Commonsense Approach to Coronary Care*. St Louis, Missouri: C.V. Mosby, 1989.

SUPPORTING THE

WHAT IS PMS?

- The majority of women suffer some premenstrual symptoms, such as fatigue, backache or headache, which are not severe enough to disrupt their lives. It is estimated that about 30% of women find symptoms so disabling that they seek medical help to cope with them.[1]
- Premenstrual syndrome (PMS) has been defined as 'distressing physical, psychological and behavioural symptoms not caused by organic disease, which regularly occur during the same phase of the menstrual cycle and which significantly regress or disappear during the remainder of the cycle'.[2]

WHY DOES PMS OCCUR?

- There are many factors implicated as triggers of PMS, although it has been pointed out that there is little evidence to support any of them.[1]
- There is a relationship between PMS and ovarian activity. Symptoms disappear in pregnancy and after the menopause but persist after hysterectomy if the ovaries are conserved. Figure 1 shows the hormone swings in the menstrual cycle: one theory is that an imbalance of the oestrogen: progesterone ratio occurs in PMS.
- Other theories include a neurotransmitter or a neuropeptide imbalance; alteration of the brain amines; fluctuating blood sugars; alterations to the immune system caused by stress; defective conversion of linoleic acids to prostaglandin E_1, resulting in an excess of prolactin and reduced vitamin B_6 intake which causes faulty co-enzyme reactions.
- It has been suggested that PMS is probably caused by a combination of these factors, and this seems to be the most helpful way to explain the aetiology of this disorder at present.

COMMON SYMPTOMS OF PMS

The most common symptoms are summarised below. Most women with PMS will have at least one symptom from each category, usually during the luteal phase of their cycle.
- **Physical symptoms:** headaches and migraines, weight gain, abdominal bloating, breast tenderness, backache, skin eruptions, hot flushes, dizziness, rhinitis, sore eyes, food cravings, changes in appetite, changes in libido.
- **Behavioural symptoms:** loss of concentration, poor work performance, avoidance of social activities, tendency to accidents, attempted suicide, violent (possibly criminal) behaviour to others
- **Psychological symptoms:** tension, apathy, irritability, depression, mood swings, anxiety, feelings of losing control, weepiness, poor self-esteem, suicidal thoughts, hostile and angry feelings.

DIAGNOSING PMS

- A daily symptom assessment diary can be helpful. The woman records all symptoms experienced during at least two menstrual cycles on each day they occur and records the date when menstruation begins and ends. In addition, women can be asked to rate the severity of symptoms.[3,4] The PMS sufferer will have symptoms of greater intensity during the premenstrual weeks. Women with menstrual distress will have symptoms present throughout the menstrual cycle, although they often increase in severity premenstrually and during menstruation.
- An alternative way of reaching a diagnosis may be to show the woman a symptom list and ask her to indicate which of them apply to her.
- Other conditions that may mimic PMS must be excluded. These include thyroid disease, anaemia, blood sugar abnormalities and other endocrine disorders.
- It is important to recognise that depression may be the underlying cause of some psychological symptoms. Depression may coexist with PMS and both conditions might need treating.
- Symptoms often start after a pregnancy or after stopping contraception. Onset may also be related to stress.

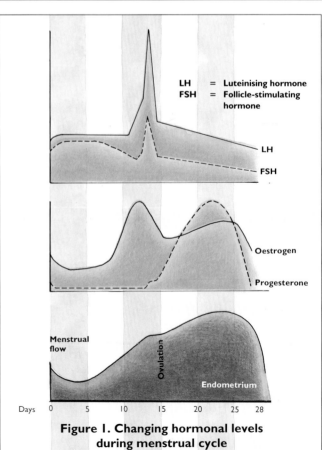

Figure 1. Changing hormonal levels during menstrual cycle

TREATING PMS

- The PMS sufferer should be the person to assess the severity of her symptoms, and treatment should be based on this assessment. Specialists in the treatment of PMS have noted that many women feel reassured after realising that they are not 'mad'. Much can be accomplished through sympathetic support in helping women to cope with their symptoms.[1,3,4]
- Difficulty in pinpointing one definite cause for PMS has led to the proliferation of a number of treatments, some hormonal and others requiring changes in diet or dietary supplements. For women who suffer from mild to moderate PMS, some changes in lifestyle and diet can be beneficial. For women whose symptoms are moderate to severe, additional hormonal treatment may be indicated.
- Treatment with progesterone, either taken orally or given as a vaginal pessary or as a suppository, has been popular, but there is some doubt about its efficacy.[3] However, it is still recommended and used by some specialists in the treatment of PMS. Other drug treatments are designed to suppress ovulation by adequate doses of oestrogen, which can now be given via oestrogen patches. Danazol will also suppress ovulation but has side-effects of nausea and dizziness. These are all drugs about which women might seek information, so it is worth looking them up if you are unfamiliar with their use.
- Most women with PMS can be helped through some simple changes to their lifestyle. Undertaking these changes themselves gives them a renewed sense of control over their symptoms. A sympathetic and non-judgemental approach to giving this information will ensure that health professionals are not seen as dismissing symptoms as trivial.
- The oral contraceptive pill is only occasionally effective in reducing symptoms of PMS, because hormone dosage levels fluctuate.

WHAT ADVICE MAY BE GIVEN?

- A study of the eating habits of women with PMS showed that they ate more refined carbohydrates, protein and dairy products than women in a control group.[1] They also ate less fibre and fewer vegetables. Caffeine can worsen anxiety and insomnia, so tea and coffee consumption should be reduced to two or three cups a day unless decaffeinated. A women with PMS should be advised to eat a diet which is high in fibre, pulses, fruit and vegetables and low in fat and animal proteins. Salt should not be added to food. Alcohol consumption should be kept low because it alters mood.
- Avoiding stressful situations during the time of the worst symptoms may prove helpful.
- Regular exercise can reduce stress and promote feelings of well-being. Yoga or t'ai chi may also be beneficial.
- It is logical that conditions which are caused by deficiencies in nutrients and amino acids could respond to treatment with them. It is known that pyridoxine (vitamin B_6) is required for many biochemical reactions in the body and that lack of it can cause an imbalance in brain amines and lead to depression. Some women have reported improvement in their PMS symptoms when they take a daily supplement of vitamin B_6. The dose should not exceed 150mg daily, as overdosage can cause peripheral neuropathy. Toxicity appears to be linked with length of treatment rather than dosage alone.
- Another food supplement which is helpful for some PMS sufferers is evening primrose oil (0.5–1g daily). It is thought to aid in the conversion of linoleic acid to gamma-linoleic acid and therefore control excessive production of prolactin, which causes depression.
- It is thought that pyridoxine and evening primrose oil are more effective if taken with other vitamin supplements, especially vitamin C, and with certain minerals.
- Magnesium is thought to alleviate breast tenderness. The dosage should be 200–300mg daily.
- Vitamin E may also be helpful in treating breast tenderness.
- Contact with a PMS sufferers support group can also be beneficial.

NOW YOU SHOULD BE ABLE TO:

- Recognise the symptoms of PMS and discuss possible causes
- Understand the rationale for treatment of PMS
- Recommend self-help measures for women with PMS.

REFERENCES
[1] Watson, N.R., Studd, J.W.W. Diagnosis and management of the premenstrual syndrome. *Update* 1991; **12**: 5.
[2] Trewinnard, K. Helping your patients to beat the premenstrual syndrome. *Horizons* 1990; **4**: 7.
[3] Magos, A.L., Studd, J.W.W. The premenstrual syndrome. In: Studd, J.W.W. (ed.). *Progress in Obstetrics and Gynaecology: Volume 4*. Edinburgh: Churchill Livingstone, 1984.
[4] Wilson, R. PMS: timing of symptoms is key to diagnosis. *Modern Medicine* 1989; **34**: 12.

FURTHER INFORMATION
National Association for Premenstrual Syndrome, PO Box 72, Sevenoaks, Kent TN13 3PS.
Premenstrual Society, PO Box 102, London SE1 7ES.

INSULIN-DEPENDENT DIABETES

WHO MAY PRESENT?

■ Insulin-dependent diabetes (IDD) can occur at any age but most commonly presents in people under 30 years. Insulin therapy would probably be initiated in hospital after diagnosis. This update concentrates on the continuing care of adults with IDD. For more information about the care of the patient with diabetes, contact your local diabetes specialist nurse.

■ Many adult patients who are stabilised on insulin therapy will be cared for by the primary health care team and should be on record as having IDD. They may not attend hospital more than once a year, so their general practice will be the source of information and follow-up. You would expect to find eight in 1,000 patients with diabetes, and of these one-third are likely to be insulin-dependent.[1]

DIAGNOSING IDD

■ The common symptoms of diabetes are well known: polydipsia, polyuria and weight loss would all indicate the possibility of diabetes. It is also important to differentiate between insulin-dependent diabetes (type I) and non-insulin-dependent diabetes (type II), and the key variables are:
— Age of onset: patients are most commonly under 30
— Speed of onset: symptoms usually occur suddenly, with rapid weight loss
— Build: those with IDD are usually thin, while 90% of patients not dependent on insulin are obese
— Tendency to ketosis: IDD patients are more prone to this.[2]

■ A urine test for the presence of glucose will be positive, and a random blood glucose measurement of 11mmol/l or above is indicative of diabetes. If the symptoms suggest IDD, test the urine for ketones, too.

■ Occasionally a person who has become diabetic will not present with the classical symptoms but with one of a number of possible complications of the disease.[3] These include:
— Skin infections, such as boils
— Leg ulcers
— Poor peripheral circulation
— Pruritis vulva or balanitis
— Dry mouth
— Excessive tiredness and loss of energy
— Deterioration of vision
— Slow-healing wounds or recurrent skin infections.

■ There is a slight predisposition for a child to develop IDD if a parent has diabetes. However, 90% of children with a diabetic parent do not develop the disease.[2]

GENERAL CONSIDERATIONS

■ The aim of management is to achieve good control of blood sugar levels. This will enable the patient to have a full and active life with as little disruption as possible. Since most people who have IDD have to control their own blood sugar levels, patient education and understanding are of paramount importance.

■ Good control of blood glucose levels is vital in preventing the long-term complications of diabetes. These include end-organ damage to the kidneys, eyes, skin and connective tissue, as well as vascular disease and neuropathies. In addition, hyper- and hypoglycaemia can occur, causing unpleasant symptoms; if untreated, both conditions are potentially fatal.

■ Insulin is now available from animal sources (beef and pork) and there is also genetically engineered so-called human insulin. There are various types of insulin prepared so that they have short, intermediate or prolonged action. Insulin is administered by subcutaneous injection, and disposable plastic syringes with attached needles are now frequently used. They can be used safely for about five injections before being discarded in accordance with local policies. Pen syringes are also gaining popularity; they give a measured dose of insulin and are easy to use.

CARE FOR THE NEWLY DIAGNOSED PATIENT

■ Although patients with type I diabetes will almost certainly be referred to hospital as a matter of urgency for stabilising blood glucose with insulin treatment, they need support and explanation from the moment diabetes is suspected.

■ Patients will probably be upset and therefore not able to remember a great deal of information, so it may be helpful to ask what they know about diabetes. This gives a chance for patients to share any fears they might have.

■ Explain what treatment is likely to be necessary, including the use of insulin and the need for dietary awareness, but do not give a detailed diet plan, as the patient will see a dietitian in hospital and conflicting information could confuse.

■ Show the patient a syringe and needle and explain that the injection is given under the skin.

■ Explain that most of the monitoring of the condition will be undertaken by the primary health care team and that a hospital stay is only required for stabilisation. If you know of diabetes shared care schemes in your area, describe how these work.

■ Be reassuring but do not be unrealistic. It is unhelpful to tell patients or relatives that 'it is nothing to worry about'.

ASPECTS OF EDUCATION

- The principles of dietary advice are that the diet should be high in fibre-rich carbohydrates, low in saturated fat, sugar and alcohol.
- People with diabetes are more susceptible to atherosclerosis and should be aware of ways in which they can minimise risks. These include stopping smoking and monitoring other risks such as hyperlipidaemia and hypertension.
- Insulin should never be adjusted on the basis of one reading only. The blood glucose levels should be monitored over two or three days to identify a pattern.
- Consistent advice must be given to people about what they should do in case of illness. They should be told to continue taking insulin, drink plenty of non-sugary fluids, test their blood sugar levels frequently to monitor control and, if the level rises above 13mmol/l, test their urine for ketones. If they are not able to eat, they should replace their normal diet with soft food or fluids.[4]
- It is vital that patients know the symptoms of hypoglycaemia. They should be told that common causes include missed meals, extra exercise and too much insulin or alcohol.

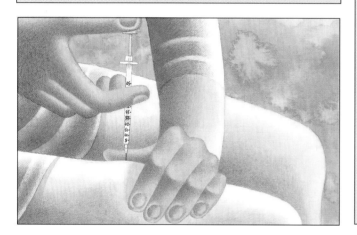

LONG-TERM CARE

- In many areas protocols for caring for the person with diabetes have been agreed between hospital and community medical and nursing personnel. You should have copies of these. Within a practice it is also a good idea to agree a protocol about who does what in giving information and in monitoring control of blood sugar and the general well-being of patients.
- It is important for practice nurses and district nurses to discuss their roles in caring for adult patients with IDD. Most will be attending the surgery for continuing monitoring of their condition at varying intervals. In addition, the district nurse may well be visiting to teach injection technique, advise about insulin storage, the disposal of syringes and needles, demonstrate blood glucose monitoring, teach about a range of health issues related to diabetes and reinforce dietary advice. If two nurses are giving conflicting advice it is confusing for patients.
- When the diabetes is stable and the patient feels confident about self-care, annual checks are adequate. Until then, the patient should be offered regular consultations.

CLINICAL PROTOCOLS 1

- Initial and continuing assessments should always include the following examinations:
—Blood pressure, usually lying and standing
—Weight and height to determine body mass index
—Urine testing for glucose, ketones and albumin (the presence of albumin could indicate renal damage)
—Plasma glucose and glycosylated haemoglobin
—Plasma lipids
—Urea and creatinine levels (possibly indicating renal damage)
—Thyroid function tests.
- Other tests which may be conducted include full blood count and erythrocyte sedimentation rate (ESR), chest X-ray and ECG. If the patient is admitted to hospital for initial treatment, these investigations will probably be carried out there.

CLINICAL PROTOCOLS 2

- At annual assessment other examinations should be added to the protocol. These are:
—Inspection of feet
—Palpation of peripheral pulses
—Assessment of sensation and reflexes
—Examination of fundi and testing of visual acuity.
- The annual review should also include:
—A recent history of the patient's health, subjective as well as objective, so that questions allow the person to voice his or her personal anxieties
—An assessment of home blood and urine glucose monitoring, with the patient demonstrating how he or she carries this out
—A discussion about diet
—Assessment of treatment and any hyper- or hypoglycaemic attacks
—Inspection of insulin sites to check for lipohypertrophy or lipoatrophy.

YOU SHOULD NOW FEEL COMPETENT TO:

- Identify your learning needs in relation to the care of the patient with IDD
- Explain the importance of coordinated care
- Take a lead in constructing a practice protocol.

REFERENCES
[1] Stilwell, B., Hobbs, R. Nursing in General Practice: Clinical Care. Oxford: Radcliffe Medical Press, 1990.
[2] Bloom, A., Ireland, J. A Colour Atlas of Diabetes. London: Wolfe Publishing, 1992.
[3] Steward, E., Oliver, J., White. M. Diabetes: Clinical Guidelines for Practice Nurses. London: RCN, 1991.
[4] Whitbourn, J. Structuring your approach. Diabetes in General Practice 1992; Spring, 5–7.

FURTHER READING
Farr, J., Watkinson, M. Diabetes: A Guide to Patient Management for Practice Nurses. Oxford: Radcliffe Medical Press, 1989.

ASSESSING WRIST AND ANKLE INJURIES

GENERAL CONSIDERATIONS

- Most people who sustain a severe injury will seek treatment at an accident and emergency department soon after the incident. Those who seek advice from a nurse or GP may have a less serious injury which has been present for 24–48 hours but which has not become less painful or swollen in that time.
- It is important to ask for a full history of the timing and nature of the injury. Some falls produce characteristic injuries, such as falling on an outstretched hand which may result in a Colles' fracture or a fracture of the scaphoid bone. Sports injuries to the ankle that occur while running may result in the rupture of a tendon. Swelling in a joint should be considered in relation to the time of the injury: immediate swelling is likely to be caused by blood leaking into and around a joint, whereas swelling that develops some hours after an injury

occurred is more likely to be caused by excessive synovial fluid.
- Ask about measures which have been taken by the patient to alleviate pain or swelling since the injury. If a joint has been rested and elevated, the swelling will be less than if the joint has been used. If the patient has recently taken an analgesic, the pain on active and passive movement will be dulled.
- Remember to ask about activities of daily living and whether the injury has been severe enough to restrict mobility or painful enough to wake the patient from sleep.
- Those who sustain sports injuries might benefit from consultation and advice at a specialised sports injuries clinic. The benefits include appropriate education to help the injured person avoid future similar injuries and advice about training the injured limb so that it regains strength.

ASSESSING INJURIES TO THE WRIST

- How did the accident occur? Was it a fall on to an outstretched hand? How long ago did it happen? How has the wrist been used since then? Has any analgesia been taken and, if so, when?
- Observe and note any swelling in the wrist. Both arms should be exposed so that there is an adequate view of the injury site and so that the size of the normal and injured sides can be compared. Then note whether there is bruising, because this could aid in the diagnosis of a fracture. (Bruising denotes bleeding into the tissues, which might be a result of a breach in the articular cartilage.)
- Test the movements in both wrists, beginning with the healthy side. Ask the patient to flex and extend the wrists, to adduct and abduct them, and observe the degree of deviation. Note if and when pain occurs, the limitations to movement and any abnormal movements. See if the patient can press together the tips of the thumb and index finger to make a circle: when the scaphoid is fractured this movement is usually painful.
- Ask the patient to make a fist or to squeeze your finger. If the patient cannot do this without pain, it is possible that the muscle contraction is causing a fractured bone to move and hence causing pain. Grip may be extremely weak or non-existent if the pain is severe.
- Palpate gently over the site of the injury to see if there is localised pain over a bone which may indicate a fracture. Feel for and listen for, but do not try to elicit, bony crepitus, which is the grinding noise made by the pieces of a broken bone.
- If the range of movements is full, there is no deformity of the joint and there is little tenderness on palpation, nor much pain on active movement even though swelling may be present, there is unlikely to be a fracture. If you are in doubt about any of these signs, seek advice from a medical practitioner.

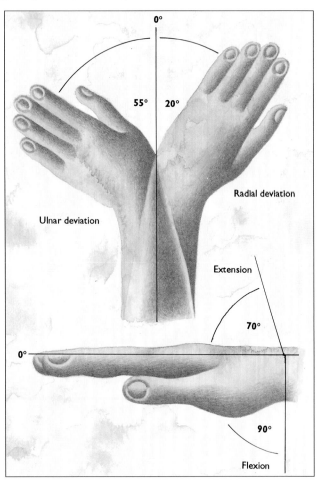

0°

55°   20°

Radial deviation

Ulnar deviation

Extension

70°

0°

90°

Flexion

TYPES OF JOINT INJURIES

■ A sprain occurs when the capsule and the synovial membrane of a joint are stretched. The synovial membrane produces excessive synovial fluid, which causes swelling. If the synovial membrane is torn, the fluid will contain some blood.

■ A strain is caused by the stretching of muscles or ligaments and may produce little or no swelling but some pain on movement.

■ A contusion is caused by an injury in which a jolt damages the two articulating surfaces of a joint which no longer move together smoothly. This results in an increase in synovial fluid within the joint capsule. Once swollen, pain on movement will not be as great as when the injury first occurred.

■ Fractures into a joint cause some bleeding into that joint, because the articular cartilage will have been torn. Swelling will occur within 20 minutes of the injury.

■ Dislocation of a joint is the complete loss of apposition of its articular surfaces. It is suspected when the bony landmarks of a joint are displaced and movement is abnormal. A fracture may be complicated by dislocation, as in Pott's fracture of the ankle.

SIGNS OF A FRACTURE

There are five cardinal signs of a fracture:

■ Loss of function: you will be testing for this when getting patients to move their wrists or ankles through the normal range of movements for that joint. This includes the ability to make a strong fist.

■ Deformity: observe for any deformity in the joint. If you are familiar with the normal bony landmarks, you will notice deformities more easily.

■ Abnormal mobility: be sure that the joint does not move, or cannot be moved, through a greater range of motion than normal. This may indicate a fracture or a ruptured tendon.

■ Localised bony tenderness: this occurs over the site of a fracture. More generalised tenderness may indicate a contusion.

■ Bony crepitus: this is when the two ends of a fractured bone rub together. No attempt should be made to produce this sign intentionally because it is extremely painful for the patient. However, you may notice it during examination.

ASSESSING THE INJURED ANKLE

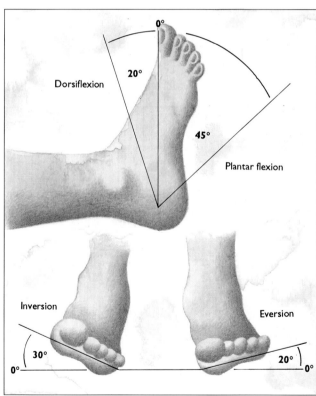

■ Begin by taking a history of the injury, including how and when it happened and whether analgesics have been taken. The ankle is a weight-bearing joint, so mobility will certainly be impaired. Ankles are particularly vulnerable to twisting injuries, which may rupture a tendon, causing considerable pain and abnormal movements of the joint.

■ Expose both legs from knee to ankle and observe for swelling and bruising. If an ankle is fractured, there could be $1/4 - 1/2$ pint loss of blood into and around the joint and the skin may be discoloured quite a way up the leg, although the bruising may not be painful away from the site of the fracture. Slight swelling of the ankle can be discerned if there is loss of the usual landmarks of the medial and/or lateral malleoli. The patient may suffer from swollen ankles for other reasons, so ask about this if both ankles appear swollen.

■ Ask the patient to move each ankle through the full normal range of movements. Note whether there is pain at any time and whether there is any deformity of the joint or abnormal movement. Can the patient wiggle the toes without pain?

■ Can the patient bear any weight on the joint? Is the toe or heel on the affected side being put to the floor or is the patient hopping? A fracture would make any weight-bearing painful.

■ Palpate the joint gently to elicit any tenderness over one spot, which could indicate a fracture.

■ If movements are full, with little pain, and there is no deformity of the ankle, the joint is probably sprained. If there is any doubt, arrange for the patient to consult a doctor.

YOU SHOULD NOW FEEL COMPETENT TO:

■ Gauge the normal range of movements in wrist and ankle
■ Watch out for the cardinal signs of a fracture
■ Be able to assess the patient presenting with a wrist or ankle injury.

Marsden, N. *Diagnosis Before First Aid.* Edinburgh: Churchill Livingstone, 1985.
Morton, P.G. *Health Assessment: A Nurse's Clinical Guide.* Springhouse, Pa.: Springhouse, 1990.

FURTHER READING
Bates, B. *A Guide to Physical Examination and History Taking.* Philadelphia, Pa.: J.B. Lippincott, 1990.

CATHETER CARE

WHEN WILL A URINARY CATHETER BE REQUIRED?

Research on 54 patients (aged 16 years and over) living in the community with long-term urinary catheters *in situ* revealed that the three most common underlying conditions were cerebrovascular/arterial disease, multiple sclerosis and paraplegia.[1] These figures would suggest that the most usual reason for long-term catheterisation is difficulty with voiding, leading either to retention of urine or to urinary incontinence.

Catheterisation may also be carried out as an emergency procedure to relieve acute retention of urine.

As a last resort, catheterisation may be used to control continence, especially if, through excoriation, the skin has broken down and there is an open wound.

Some patients now achieve continence through intermittent catheterisation performed by the patient or by a carer.

GENERAL INFORMATION

It is accepted that most patients who have a urinary catheter *in situ* for 10 days or longer will develop bacteriuria.[2] This leads to catheter blockage, which is a common complication of long-term catheter usage.

Factors associated with catheter blockage include the pH of the urine — which tends to be alkaline in patients with a blockage — and the presence of the proteus organism in the urine. It is thought that this chain of events leads to the build-up of deposits around the catheter tip and causes blockage.[1]

Blockage can cause leakage.

A small research study, based in the community, showed that a hydrogel-coated catheter can be left *in situ* for longer than a silicone-coated catheter, without the associated problems of blockage and leakage and with no loss of comfort for the patient.[2] The study's author makes the point that nurses in the community should be aware of the different catheters available for use and should look analytically at the catheters they use.

The use of oral ascorbic acid and bladder wash-outs are two ways of acidifying urine. However, there is no research evidence to support the effectiveness of either of these two techniques.

The long-term use of antibiotic therapy to prevent urinary tract infections is now discouraged. Antibiotics are recommended when patients present with symptoms of urinary tract infection.

CARING FOR A PATIENT WITH AN INDWELLING CATHETER

Patients with indwelling catheters will be at different stages of dependency: some will be ambulant, others confined to bed or wheelchair. Nursing intervention required will depend on the patient's independence.

The primary objectives of caring for a patient with an indwelling catheter are to promote the comfort and well-being of the patient and to prevent complications from the presence of the catheter. The main complications are likely to be blockages and infections.

DAILY CATHETER CARE

Cleaning the meatus and the perineal area is accepted as an important part of catheter care because it is thought to help prevent infection. Research has not demonstrated any link between meatal cleaning and the prevention of bacteriuria.[3] This may be because the nursing techniques are not correctly performed, and an understanding of the principles of asepsis and prevention of cross-infection may promote better technique than simply learning procedures.[3]

If patients are ambulant, they should be encouraged to manage their catheter hygiene themselves and, by doing so, reduce the risk of cross-infection from other patients.

The perineal area can be cleaned with soap and water, and care should be taken to clean from the front to the back of the perineum. The swab or cloth used for cleaning must not be used on a possibly contaminated area and then around the urinary meatus. In practice, this means that swabs are used once only to wipe from the front of the perineum to the back. They are then discarded. If a cloth is used, a separate area of the cloth must be used for each stroke. If soap and water is used for cleaning, the swabs or cloth used do not have to be sterile.

If it is decided that sterile swabs and an antiseptic are to be used to clean the perineum, there should be consistency in the maintenance of asepsis. This means that the swabs should be sterile and should be placed only on a sterile surface before use. The lotion to be used should be placed in a sterile container. Swabs must be used once only from front to back.

Effective hand-washing techniques will reduce the risk of infection and should be practised whether or not gloves are worn. If patients are undertaking catheter care themselves, they, too, must be taught how to wash and dry their hands thoroughly. Hand-washing is as important when catheter care is part of the daily hygiene routine and done with soap and water as it is when an aseptic technique is used.

It is generally accepted that the perineal area should be cleaned twice a day and after every bowel movement.

Powders and lotions should not be used after cleaning because they can trap organisms in the area.

CARE OF THE DRAINAGE BAG

Emptying the drainage bag provides opportunities for bacterial contamination and so must be carried out with attention to the prevention of infection.

Hands should be thoroughly washed before emptying the bag.

The tap should be cleaned before opening and again afterwards.

The bag should be emptied into a container which is discarded or thoroughly washed and dried. The container should not be used for more than one patient.

The tap should not touch the sides of the container, the urine or the floor. It should be washed and dried after use and securely closed.

The bag must be at a lower level than the bladder to prevent urine seeping back into the bladder. It is important to explain this to patients who are self-caring and to tell them to clamp the tubing if the bag has to be lifted up for any reason.

If the bag has to be changed, a hygienic technique must be used so that no part of the tubing becomes contaminated.

The frequency of emptying of the bag will depend on individual patients' needs.

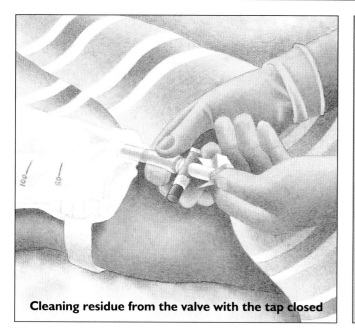

Cleaning residue from the valve with the tap closed

PROMOTING PATIENT COMFORT

The patient's comfort can be ensured by providing a catheter of the right size, maintaining the correct balloon size and by confident and gentle handling of the catheter. Educating the patient about the function of a catheter and how it should be cared for can reduce anxiety and promote a positive attitude to living with an indwelling catheter.

While size selection has been found to be appropriate in most cases, balloon size has been found to be too large in as many as 72% of patients.[3] A balloon infill volume of 10ml will generally provide adequate drainage and cause less discomfort to the patient than the more usual 30ml infill volume.

The balloon can also cause irritation and discomfort if it pulls on the internal sphincter. To prevent this, the catheter tubing can be anchored to the thigh, leaving some slack between the place where the catheter tubing is attached and the urinary meatus.

OTHER NURSING CARE POINTS

A generous fluid intake should be encouraged. It should be explained to the patient why this is necessary and an intake of 2500–3000ml daily is recommended. Explanation to patients and carers about how much this represents in terms of cups or glasses will help them gauge the amount they are drinking.

When patients are ambulant they should be encouraged to move about. This helps promote adequate emptying of the bladder through gravity and thereby prevent stagnation of urine. It also increases the independence and well-being of the patient.

Patients should be encouraged to report any changes in their condition to the nurse or carer. These include burning sensations around the catheter, leakage of urine or a feeling of feverishness. The nurse, or the self-caring patient, should note if the urine becomes cloudy or strong-smelling. All of these changes can be signs and symptoms of urinary tract infection or catheter blockage.

The catheter tubing leading to the bag must not be allowed to become kinked. If it does, it can cause the tubing to separate and increase the risk of bacterial contamination.

AFTER READING THIS YOU SHOULD:

Understand the importance of monitoring practice in the light of current research

Have revised some of the techniques of catheter care

Have reflected on the importance of patient education and the promotion of well-being for those with catheters.

REFERENCES
[1] Kohler-Ockmore, J. Chronic urinary catheter blockage. *Nursing Standard* 1991; **5**: 44, 26–28.
[2] Bull, H. Long-term catheterisation. *Journal of District Nursing* 1990; December, 4-7.
[3] Crow, R., Chapman, R., Roe, B. et al. *A Study of Patients with an Indwelling Urethral Catheter and Related Nursing Practice.* Guildford: Nursing Practice Research Unit, University of Surrey, 1986.

ASSESSING PATIENTS WITH COLDS AND FLU

WHO MAY PRESENT

- An adult who has a fever and feels generally off-colour
- An adult with persistent symptoms of a cold.

GENERAL CONSIDERATIONS

- Many people suffer from colds and what is often termed 'flu' in the winter. For most people, sensible symptomatic treatment at home for a few days is all that is needed before they feel better. Others will seek the advice of a nurse or doctor for a variety of reasons:
  — A 'sick note' is needed for work
  — A person needs to be confirmed as ill so that he or she may feel justified in ceasing normal daily activity and where the individual wants to have a period of rest from his or her usual role as carer or worker
  — Symptoms are unusual or unexpected
  — Symptoms have persisted longer than expected
  — Being accustomed to consulting a doctor or nurse about every minor condition. This can be reinforced if anti-biotics have been prescribed frequently. It is important to find out exactly why patients are attending for advice about something that they term as a cold or flu.
- There are many viruses which can cause coryzal symptoms, sore throat, fever and coughs. The most common cause of a cold (coryza) is one of the hundred or more strains of the rhinovirus.
- There are three types of influenza virus, known as A, B and C. Infection by influenza A virus is most common and causes more severe illness than B or C. Influenza A virus undergoes changes in its surface antigens from time to time, and immunity is not transferred to the new strain of influenza A virus. Some results of these antigenic changes have included the Asian flu, which is no longer circulating, and the Hong Kong and red flus, which are both still around.
- The adenovirus and the echovirus cause similar symptoms to the influenza virus, but the patient is usually less ill and recovers more quickly.
- Occasionally there are major epidemics of influenza, such as in the winter of 1989 (Fig. 1) and those people who are particularly vulnerable to serious complications following influenza, such as the elderly or those with a chronic illness, should be immunised against the prevailing strains. Present vaccines provide 90% immunity for one year.
- Children, pregnant women and those who are elderly or vulnerable to infection should always be assessed by a medical practitioner.

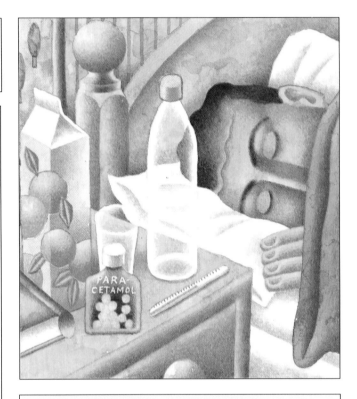

TAKING A HISTORY

- Be sure to ask open-ended questions when you are taking a history. This means that you do not ask questions that invite a 'yes' or 'no' answer but, rather, ones that encourage a patient to provide as much information as he or she can. This is important because it will help you to identify your patient's most urgent needs. Helpful, open-ended questions in a consultation might include 'Tell me about this illness. What sort of symptoms do you have?' or 'What sort of job do you have and what does it involve?' Not only will you find out about the illness but also about whether the patient has a hard manual job or works outdoors and/or needs a certificate to be absent from work.
- You need to ensure that you obtain the following information:
  — When the illness started and whether the onset was sudden or gradual
  — Whether anyone in the patient's household or workplace has similar symptoms
  — What the symptoms are
  — What the patient has been doing about the illness, such as staying in bed, taking paracetamol or other over-the-counter remedies, staying off work and how effective the patient's treatment is at alleviating the symptoms.

CLINICAL SIGNS AND SYMPTOMS OF A COLD

- A cold is often preceded by a sore throat.
- The patient may report that he or she has been in contact with someone who has had a cold. The incubation period for rhinovirus is one to two days and for para-influenza viruses, which also cause coryzal symptoms, five to six days.
- Fever is usually slight, and the patient often does not feel ill enough to stay in bed.
- Coryzal symptoms, that is, runny nose and eyes, last about three days.
- An uncomplicated recovery usually takes place between five and 10 days after the onset of symptoms.

CLINICAL SIGNS AND SYMPTOMS OF INFLUENZA

- One of the most common features of the influenza virus is that it spreads rapidly among members of the same household, and this is a useful clinical pointer to the disease.
- The onset is usually sudden. The temperature rises from the early stages of the illness and may be the first sign of the virus. A high fever may persist from the first to the fourth day of the illness.
- A dry cough develops early in the illness and becomes productive any time from the second to the fourth day.
- Retrosternal pain on coughing is fairly common and suggests a characteristic tracheitis.
- Headache, backache and muscular aches and pains are experienced by a third to a half of people with influenza. These symptoms often accompany a high fever.
- The throat may be sore, perhaps through coughing.

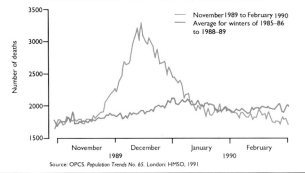

Figure 1. Daily deaths in November 1989 to March 1990, compared with the daily average for the same days in the winters of 1985–86 to 1988–89, Great Britain

— November 1989 to February 1990
— Average for winters of 1985–86 to 1988–89

Number of deaths: 3500, 3000, 2500, 2000, 1500

November 1989, December, January 1990, February

Source: OPCS. *Population Trends No. 65.* London: HMSO, 1991

ASSESSING SYMPTOMS

When you should refer to a doctor:
- If the acute febrile illness has been present for longer than four days
- If the patient is elderly, bed-bound or vulnerable to infection
- If the patient is the only member of a household with these symptoms, particularly if recently arrived or returned from a tropical country
- If a fever and cough persist with purulent sputum
- If the patient is a child and is the only member of a household with a febrile illness
- If the patient complains of back or neck stiffness which is persistent and painful. This may indicate meningitis or encephalitis.

DISEASES THAT MAY BE CONFUSED WITH INFLUENZA

- The common cold may also give rise to febrile illness and sore throat but usually causes a runny nose and eyes. The patient is not, as a rule, ill enough to stay in bed and the fever is not as high as that caused by influenza.
- Bronchitis and tracheitis cause cough and fever. These illnesses are often preceded by coryzal symptoms and will probably not be a household epidemic.
- Infections with other viruses, such as adenovirus or echovirus, can cause symptoms similar to those of influenza but not usually as severe.
- Tonsillitis can cause a sore throat and fever.

ADVICE TO GIVE TO THE PATIENT WITH INFLUENZA

- Stay in bed while the fever lasts and resume normal activity slowly.
- Take paracetamol for pain and fever.
- Drink adequate amounts of fluids, including fruit juices and water, to maintain hydration and keep fever down.
- Try to keep the temperature in the room steady. This can prevent secondary chest infection or hypothermia in an inactive elderly person.
- Report any worsening of symptoms to the nurse or the doctor. These might include a rising fever, a cough, severe neck stiffness or headache. Convalescence is gradual, beginning around the fourth day of the illness. If deterioration occurs after this time, it is suggestive of a secondary bacterial infection.

NOW YOU SHOULD FEEL COMPETENT TO:

- Take a relevant history from a patient who is complaining of the cold/influenza symptoms
- Understand the importance of the reported symptoms
- Know when referral to a doctor is necessary
- Offer advice about management of colds and influenza.

FURTHER READING
Hodgkin, K. *Towards Earlier Diagnosis: A Guide to Primary Care.* Edinburgh: Churchill Livingstone, 1985

Barbara Stilwell, BSocSci, RGN, RHV, is principal lecturer in health and community studies at the Institute of Advanced Nursing Education, RCN, London, and a nurse practitioner.

NEXT MONTH: SYRINGE DRIVERS

ASSESSING THE ADULT WITH CONSTIPATION

WHO MAY PRESENT?

Constipation is not a common presenting symptom, although many people of all ages express concern about their bowel habits.[1] There are, however, certain times in life when constipation is more likely to seem a problem:

■ In infancy, when parents may become concerned if the child's bowel habits change or stool consistency changes
■ In the older child, when parents may attribute a range of symptoms to constipation
■ In pregnancy and during menstruation, when a combination of hormonal and other physiological changes affect the bowel[2]
■ In old age, when bowel motility slows down and, in addition, diet may lack fibre.

The presentation of constipation as a troublesome symptom by someone in middle age should always be taken seriously. While it may be due to a number of innocuous factors, it may also signify a change of bowel habit suggestive of large bowel cancer.[1] Adequate history-taking and appropriate referral are therefore vital.

This Update deals only with assessing the adult who complains of constipation.

WHAT IS CONSTIPATION?

The term may be used to describe a number of symptoms, including infrequent bowel action, hard stools or difficulty in passing faeces. Cummings[2] has described five factors indicative of constipation:

■ The amount of stool passed: people are often aware when the amount of stool passed decreases.
■ Stool consistency: faeces are usually soft in consistency, with a characteristic shape. Constipation is likely to result in hard pellet-shaped stools.
■ Frequency of defecation: Morrell[1] cites a study which showed that 99% of nearly 1500 people questioned had a bowel action within the range of three times daily to three times weekly. As the range of normal is so wide, it is important to clarify what has been the change in frequency of bowel action when a patient complains of constipation.
■ Discomfort and straining: constipation is often associated with pain on defecation which may be due either to low abdominal colicky pain prior to defecation or to soreness around the anus because of anal fissure or haemorrhoids. If patients have to spend more than 10 minutes on the toilet to defecate, this is indicative of constipation.
■ Transit time from mouth to anus: in constipation this is usually greater than five days. However, without hospital investigation it is impossible to measure accurately.

CAUSES OF CONSTIPATION

■ Physiologically, there are two reasons why constipation may occur:
— If there is insufficient material in the bowel to ensure normal motility
— If there is obstruction or impairment of normal neuromuscular activity in the bowel or interruption of the recto-anal defecatory reflex mechanism.
■ There will be insufficient material in the bowel when there is inadequate dietary intake of fibre and starch. Fibre and starch are necessary in the bowel to stimulate bacterial growth through fermentation, which creates gas. Water is retained in undigested fibre, and it is the bacteria, undigested material, water and gas that create stool bulk. Slimming diets deficient in fibre and starch may cause constipation, as will persistent anorexia. Patients on gluten-free diets may also suffer from constipation.
■ Neuromuscular activity in the bowel can be impaired by certain drugs, including some analgesics, antacids containing aluminium, anti-depressives, some anti-hypertensive drugs and iron.
■ Cerebrovascular accidents, spinal cord injuries and pelvic surgery may all result in disturbance of the bowel's normal motor activity.
■ Recto-anal reflexes may be affected by childbirth and may be altered in elderly people. This leads to outlet obstruction syndrome where there is no coordination of the defecatory mechanism.
■ A combination of factors may give rise to constipation in certain conditions, including hypothyroidism, hypercalcaemia, diabetes, depression, pregnancy and menstruation.
■ Painful conditions of the rectum and anus, which cause the patient to avoid defecation, can lead to constipation. Ignoring the need to defecate, for whatever reason, will have the same result.
■ Irritable bowel syndrome is encountered twice as often in women and causes constipation, diarrhoea and pain in the descending colon. Stools are often pellet-shaped and hard. It is thought to be associated with abnormal colonic motility and with psychological factors.
■ Diverticular disease may cause constipation.
■ Commonly encountered causes of constipation may be a change in diet, because of holidays or travel, or periods of inactivity. It is uncertain why these lifestyle changes should have this effect.
■ Constipation, especially if it alternates with diarrhoea, may be one symptom of large bowel cancer. In elderly and middle-aged people, a careful history must be taken and a thorough examination made to exclude this diagnosis.

TAKING A HISTORY

- The key points to clarify are:
- How is the person defining constipation? Is it related to the frequency of defecation, to consistency of stools or to pain or excessive straining on passing a stool?
- How long has this symptom been present? Has it ever occurred before?
- Is there any diarrhoea? Does it alternate with constipation?
- Have laxatives been taken?
- How much dietary fibre is consumed? Has there been a recent change in diet?
- Have there been any recent lifestyle changes, such as travel, ceasing exercising or going on a diet?
- Is there any link with pregnancy or menstruation?
- What drugs (other than laxatives) have been taken? For how long? (Check whether constipation is a side-effect.)
- It is helpful to make a careful assessment of the dietary intake of fibre. Asking what the person normally has for breakfast is useful, because it is then that most people eat cereal fibres. Ask about consumption of bread and about fruit and vegetables. Remember to ask if there have been recent changes to the amount of fibre eaten daily.
- Clarify the use of laxatives. Some people have unrealistic expectations of bowel habits and may be dependent on increasing doses for bowel movements.
- Observe the overall appearance of the person. Does he or she look as though there has been recent weight loss? Are there any characteristic signs of myxoedema? Does the person appear depressed? Ask about general health status.
- Remember to ask about stool consistency and whether there is ever blood or slime present in the motion. This may indicate the presence of a cancer or other bowel disease and warrants further investigation.

THE DIGESTIVE SYSTEM

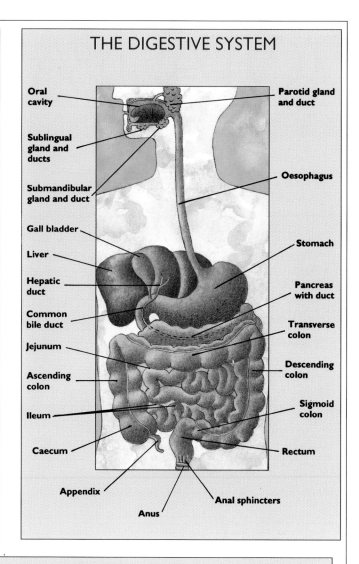

ASSESSING THE SITUATION

- To treat constipation effectively requires a firm diagnosis of its cause. Any patient who describes constipation as a new symptom which cannot be attributed to a change in diet or lifestyle requires an abdominal and rectal examination.
- Referral to a physician is always indicated in the following situations:
  - The constipation represents a change in normal bowel habits
  - The constipation alternates with diarrhoea
  - There is blood and/or slime in the stool
  - There is accompanying abdominal pain or vomiting.

- Habitual constipation may be a result of laxative abuse or poor dietary intake of fibre. If organic disease is excluded, advice about increasing dietary fibre can be given. The most effective way to do this is to increase the intake of cereals by consuming more 100% wholewheat bread (six slices a day), a wholewheat breakfast cereal or one with added bran, as well as generally eating more high-fibre foods, more fruit and vegetables and maintaing an adequate fluid intake.
- Obviously any drugs which may be implicated as a cause of constipation should be reassessed after consultation with the prescribing physician.

NOW YOU SHOULD BE ABLE TO:

- Discuss the causes of constipation in an adult
- Take an appropriate history
- Refer appropriately to a physician for further investigation.

REFERENCES
[1] Morrell, D. The patient complaining of constipation. In: Cormack, J. M., Morrell, D. (eds). *A Handbook of Primary Medical Care*. Kingston upon Thames: Kluwer Publishing, 1982.
[2] Cummings, J. Constipation: investigation and management. *Update* 1989; **39**: 1, 22–33.

TOTAL PARENTERAL

WHO MAY NEED TOTAL PARENTERAL NUTRITION?

Anyone (adult or child) who has a functional impairment of the gastrointestinal tract which makes oral food intake impracticable may require short- or long-term total parenteral nutrition (TPN). These patients will include:
■ Those with conditions that interfere with the absorption of nutrients, such as short bowel syndrome, Crohn's disease, enteric fistulas, radiation enteritis or congenital malformations
■ Those who have persistent vomiting or diarrhoea owing to chemotherapy or radiation
■ Those with AIDS-related diarrhoea
■ Those with mesenteric vascular thrombosis, when resection of a large area of gangrenous bowel may be necessary.

WHAT IS TOTAL PARENTERAL NUTRITION?

■ TPN provides all nutritional requirements intravenously, usually via a central venous line. The purpose of doing this is to bypass a non-functioning gut and allow nutrients to be absorbed directly into the venous system.
■ Parenteral nutrition can also be administered via the peripheral veins, but the solutions used have to be isotonic (that is, of the same concentration as the one they are to be mixed with — in this case blood). Around 2000 kilocalories can be provided via the peripheral route, by using lipid emulsions, but for parenteral nutrition lasting longer than five days the central venous route is more commonly preferred. This is because a central venous line allows concentrated liquids (hypertonic) to be diluted rapidly into the large blood volume in the superior vena cava. In addition, problems of thrombo-phlebitis of peripheral vessels are avoided, and patients have a once-only insertion of the central venous line which they can learn to manage themselves and which therefore gives them more independence, as well as freedom of movement.[1,2]
■ Solutions to be infused in TPN are individually tailored for each person's nutritional requirements. They will always contain seven essential ingredients: water, protein, carbohydrate, fat, electrolytes, vitamins and trace elements. The solution is commonly made up as a three-litre bag of fluid.
■ The solution is usually infused overnight using a pump to control the rate of infusion. If the infusion rate is irregular, if it is stopped or started too quickly or if the pump suddenly fails, there can be wild fluctuations in blood sugar, which can cause significant hypo- or hyperglycaemia.
■ Patients on TPN at home will be taught in hospital to care for the central venous line using an aseptic technique. They will be able to set up the infusion, mix additives in the TPN fluid and connect themselves to the infusion.

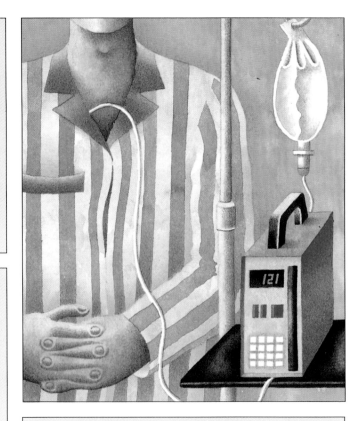

GENERAL CONSIDERATIONS

■ About 100 people in the UK are currently being nutritionally maintained on TPN at home.[3] In 1989 researchers interviewed 30 people receiving TPN and found their ages ranged from 17 to 63 years, one-third were employed and just over one-third felt able to lead a normal life.[4]
■ A Canadian research project examined the psychological and social reactions of patients who were receiving TPN at home on a permanent or semi-permanent basis. It was found that considerable psychological adjustment was needed by patients and by their families. Depression and grief were experienced by patients who had to adjust to the permanent loss of normal eating patterns. Marital and sexual relationships may be strained because of altered body image and feelings that the person receiving TPN is in some way a 'freak'.[5]
■ Patients who are to receive TPN at home will be taught the practical techniques they require to maintain this system before discharge from a specialist nutrition unit. It is important for the community nurse to remember, however, that the research evidence suggests that some patients and their families require continuing psychological, and possibly educational, support. For this reason, a nurse involved in the care of someone on TPN should be aware of the need to maintain contact with patients and their carers, although they may appear to need little practical help.

NURSING CONSIDERATIONS

■ Patients who are to receive TPN will be well established on their regime by the time they return home. The involvement of the community nurse in care will depend on the availability of a specialist nurse who, in most cases, will continue to provide care and advice. However, it is reassuring for patients to know that their local team of GP and community nurses are familiar with the regime and are able to give immediate practical help and long-term support, encouragement and advice as necessary.

■ The care of patients who have a central venous line is discussed on page 2. Refer to this information if necessary. Problems with infection, catheter occlusion and air embolus can all occur.

■ Problems specific to the care of patients receiving TPN include the following:

— Monitoring for glucose intolerance must be done by testing the urine for glycosuria twice daily. If this occurs, blood sugar levels must be monitored (initially using reagent sticks). If blood sugar levels remain high, insulin may be given (added to the solution). Provided that the TPN solution infusion rate is carefully regulated, beginning slowly, hyperglycaemia can be avoided. Hypoglycaemia may occur if the infusion is stopped too suddenly.

— Electrolyte balance must be carefully monitored and is usually checked by blood test. Twently-four-hour urine collection may be required for the same reason.

— Fluid balance can be measured by intake and output charts and by monitoring weight and signs of overload, such as oedema.

— In patients with compromised respiratory function TPN can lead to respiratory distress.

PSYCHOSOCIAL CONSIDERATIONS

■ Interrupted sleep patterns, caused by nocturnal polyuria, can result from the large amount of liquid used in the TPN solution. Patients on long-term TPN report that they become used to getting up during the night and fall asleep quickly afterwards. A daytime feeding regime is possible but interrupts normal daily activities, and this may be even more unacceptable. However, the nocturnal routine can cause fatigue and the patient may need a nap during the day, which increases the feeling of 'being ill'.

■ Anxiety about the equipment and the TPN procedures may occur. The nurse has to be aware of the importance of educating not only the patient but also the family in handling the equipment and in what to do if something goes wrong. It is also reassuring if the patient is in touch with others who are having TPN .

■ Depression is common. The patient may grieve for the rituals associated with eating. Sharing meals is often an important occasion, and many festivals are built around meals. Moreover, patients who have lost most of their bowel may feel as though they are no longer whole people, and extensive scarring, or even the presence of a central venous line, can cause an alteration of body image. It is important for the nurse to understand the process and to help the patient come to terms with loss.

■ Impairment of sexual function may occur. This can be caused by a fear of dislodging or damaging the central venous line or through altered body image. Discussing this issue with patients and their partners may allow fears and anxieties to be shared.

■ Any family supporting a member with a condition requiring special routines and procedures begins to function differently. Communication may be a problem if family members suppress their anger or other emotions in order to protect each other. While the nurse may not have the skills to help families deal with such dysfunction, it is vital to the quality of all their lives that they can receive appropriate help from a trained counsellor and that the nurse can recognise when this help might be required.

NOW YOU SHOULD BE AWARE OF:

■ The indications for TPN
■ How TPN is organised for the patient at home
■ The physical and psychosocial nursing needs likely to arise for the patient on TPN.

REFERENCES
[1] Worthington, P., Wagner, B. Total parenteral nutrition. *Nursing Clinics of North America* 1989; **24:** 2, 355–371.
[2] Michie, B. Making sense of total parenteral nutrition. *Nursing Times* 1988; **84:** 20, 46–47.
[3] Lennard-Jones, J.E., Wood, S. The organisation of intravenous feeding at home. *Health Trends* 1985; **17:** 73–75.
[4] Malons, M. Home parenteral nutrition: effect on patients' lifestyle. *Clinical Nutrition* 1989; **8:** 11–13.
[5] Price, B., Levine, E. Permanent total parenteral nutrition: psychological and social responses of the early stages. *Journal of Parenteral and Enteral Nutrition* 1979; **3:** 2, 48–52.

■ Acknowledgement is made to Jo Gibson at the Specialist Nutrition Unit, Hope Hospital, Salford, for help in preparing these pages.

Barbara Stilwell, BSocSci, RGN, RHV, is principal lecturer at the Institute of Advanced Nursing Education, RCN, London, and a nurse practitioner.